REVERSE DIABETES

A GUIDE TO TREATING AND REVERSING DIABETES
WITH DIET AND A PROVEN CURE PLAN TO LOWER
YOUR BLOOD SUGAR

Descrierea CIP a Bibliotecii Naționale a României
BARNETT, TONY
  Reverse diabetes : a guide to treating and reversing diabetes with diet and a proven cure plan to lower your blood sugar / by Tony Barnett. - București : My Ebook, 2018
    ISBN 978-606-983-611-8
616

REVERSE DIABETES

A GUIDE TO TREATING AND REVERSING DIABETES WITH DIET AND A PROVEN CURE PLAN TO LOWER YOUR BLOOD SUGAR

My Ebook Publishing House
Bucharest, 2018

CONTENTS

INTRODUCTION

I want to use this medium to thank and congratulate you for purchasing this book **"Reverse Diabetes: A Guide To Treating And Reversing Diabetes With Diet And A Proven Cure Plan To Lower Your Blood Sugar."**

Doctors, dietitians, and patients essentially take after the *tapping*: diabetes implies high blood sugars and controls it with eating regimen, exercise, and pharmaceuticals. On the off chance that one medication does not work, change to another, or include another. They all keep on chasing blood sugars like a wild goose pursue. At last, everybody is by all accounts baffled.

The motivation behind composing this book is to furnish you with logical and additionally down to earth information about diabetes: what works and what does not and why. At that point, you can utilize this data to take part in a meaningful discussion with your doctor and assume the responsibility for your diabetes.

Thanks again for buying this book and I hope you enjoy it.

This document is geared towards providing exact and reliable information in regards to the topic and issue covered. The publication is sold with the idea that the publisher is not required to render accounting, officially permitted, or otherwise, qualified services. If advice is necessary, legal or professional, a practiced individual in the profession should be ordered.

- From a Declaration of Principles which was accepted and approved equally by a Committee of the American Bar Association and a Committee of Publishers and Associations.

In no way is it legal to reproduce, duplicate, or transmit any part of this document in either electronic means or in printed format. Recording of this publication is strictly prohibited and any storage of this document is not allowed unless with written permission from the publisher. All rights reserved.

The information provided herein is stated to be truthful and consistent, in that any liability, in terms of inattention or otherwise, by any usage or abuse of any policies, processes, or directions contained within is the solitary and utter responsibility of the recipient reader. Under no circumstances will any legal responsibility or blame be held against the publisher for any reparation, damages, or monetary loss due to the information herein, either directly or indirectly.

Respective authors own all copyrights not held by the publisher.

The information herein is offered for informational purposes solely, and is universal as so. The presentation of the information is without contract or any type of guarantee assurance.

The trademarks that are used are without any consent, and the publication of the trademark is without permission or backing by the trademark owner. All trademarks and brands within this book are for clarifying purposes only and are the owned by the owners themselves, not affiliated with this document.

CHAPTER ONE

WHAT IS DIABETES?

Diabetes mellitus ordinarily alluded to as diabetes, is a group of metabolic anarchy in which there are high glucose levels over a longer period. Diabetes is suspected to either the pancreas not delivering enough insulin or the cells of the body not reacting legitimately to the insulin produced.

In simple English, Diabetes is the condition that outcomes from the absence of insulin in a man's blood, or when their body has an issue utilizing the insulin it produces (Insulin protection). There are different sorts of diabetes, similar to diabetes insipidus. Be that as it may, when individuals say "diabetes," they mean diabetes mellitus.

Glucose isn't general sugar that is accessible in stores and grocery stores. Glucose is a natural starch that our bodies use as a wellspring of vitality. The sort of sugar sold in general stores is called sucrose and is very different from glucose. High centralizations of glucose can be found in soda pops and fruits.

The glucose level in the blood is controlled by a few hormones (chemicals in your body that send messages to different cells). The glucose is utilized by cells for energy. Additional glucose that isn't required immediately is put away in a few cells as glycogen. When you are not eating, cells separate glycogen into glucose to use as energy.

However, humans aren't the only living thing that experiencing the ill effects of diabetes, even dogs too. Diabetes in these creatures has a large number of indistinguishable causes from it does in people – in particular, innate qualities, eating routine, and absence of activity, their odds of diabetes soar with each additional tick of the scale. Like people, they require insulin to keep up their wellbeing. There are both oral and injectable insulin solutions accessible to creatures, yet canines usually don't react to oral insulin. Little puppies more often than not require around two shots every day, while bigger ones can typically get by on one. Also, as you can envision, this can get, exceptionally costly

The number of individuals with diabetes has almost quadrupled since 1980. The disease's predominance is expanding around the world, especially in the under-developed nations. The causes are perplexing, yet the ascent is expected to some degree to increments in the magnitude of individuals who are overweight, incorporating an expansion in corpulence, and in a far-reaching absence of physical movement.

History Of Diabetes

Diabetes has been a significant torment for mankind from time immemorial. It is broadly described in antiquated Egyptian manuscripts dating as far back as 1550 B.C. Initially; the infection was to some degree uncommon. While the pyramids were being paved simultaneously, there weren't any 24-hour donut establishments, and quite a good number of people tried subsistence methods to slim down.

The primary clinical description of diabetes was given by the Ancient Greek doctor "Aretaeus of Cappadocia" who additionally noticed a good measure of pee which went through the kidneys."

Diabetes seems to have been a capital punishment in the antiquated time. Famous Greek physician "Hippocrates" didn't mention it, which may demonstrate that he felt the malady was bleak. "Aretaeus" attempted to treat it, however, couldn't give a decent conjecture, so he, therefore, concluded that "life (with diabetes) is short, disturbing and painful.

In medieval Persia, Avicenna (980– 1037) gave a detailed account on diabetes mellitus in The Canon of Medicine, "portraying the unusual hunger and the fall of sexual capacities," and he recorded the sweet taste of diabetic pee. Like Aretaeus before him, Avicenna had a singular headway with superficial essential and optional diabetes. He likewise depicted diabetic gangrene and treated diabetes utilizing a blend of lupine, Trigonella (fenugreek), and zedoary seed, which creates an effective diminishment in the discharge of sugar, a treatment which is as yet recommended in present day times. Avicenna likewise depicted diabetes insipidus precisely out of the blue; however, it was significantly later that Thomas Willis separated it from diabetes mellitus in a part of his book

Pharmaceutical rationalize

In spite of the fact that diabetes has been perceived since artifact, and medications of different viability have been known in various districts since the **Middle Ages**, and in the legend for any longer, pathogenesis of diabetes has just been seen tentatively since around 1900. A viable treatment was only created after the Canadians Frederick Banting, and Charles Best initially utilized insulin in 1921 and 1922.

CHAPTER TWO
TYPES AND SYMPTOMS OF DIABETES

Types of Diabetes

Pre-diabetes: Pre-diabetes is the prototype before diabetes mellitus in which not the majority of the indications required to analyze diabetes are available, yet glucose is somewhat high. This stage is frequently alluded to as the "hazy area, and it's for the most part connected with corpulence (particularly stomach or instinctive weight), dyslipidemia with high triglycerides as well as low HDL cholesterol, and hypertension. It is subsequently a metabolic diathesis or Syndrome, and it more often than includes no manifestations and just high glucose as the sole sign.

Type 1 diabetes mellitus: This kind of diabetes mellitus happens when the pancreas that makes insulin is destroyed by the individual's particular resistant framework. At the point when the pancreas does not produce insulin, glucose – sugar – in the blood can't get into the parts of the body that need sugar to live. To live, a man with Type 1 diabetes must take insulin for whatever remains of their life. They have to check their glucose level all the time, frequently, commonly every day. Type 1 diabetes happens more often than not in more youthful individuals, be that as it may, it can happen in grown-ups, in spite of the fact that this is considerably less normal. Around 1 out of each ten individuals with diabetes has Type 1 Diabetes.

Type 2 diabetes mellitus: Type 2 diabetes mellitus is different from Type 1 diabetes. In Type 2 diabetes, the person makes insulin, however, either the insulin does not work in that individual's body as it should, or they don't produce enough insulin to process the glucose. At the point when insulin does not function as it should, glucose (sugar) in the blood can't get into the parts of the body that need sugar. Type 2 kind of diabetes happens more often than not in an overweight seasoned individual.

Gestational diabetes: Gestational diabetes mellitus is more like Type 2 diabetes. It happens to a few ladies when they are pregnant which is as a result of any level of glucose intolerance when firstly acknowledged amid pregnancy. This classification applies whether insulin or just eating regimen adjustment is utilized for treatment and regardless of whether the condition continues after pregnancy. It doesn't reject the likelihood that unrecognized glucose bigotry may have preceded or started correspondingly with the pregnancy.

Steroid-induced diabetes:_ This kind of diabetes is a therapeutic term alluding to delayed hyperglycemia because of glucocorticoid therapy for another restorative condition. It is ordinarily, however not generally, a transient condition.

The widely accepted glucocorticoids which cause steroid diabetes are prednisolone and dexamethasone given fundamentally in "pharmacologic dosage" for a considerable length of time. Ordinary medicinal conditions in which steroid diabetes emerges amid high-measurement glucocorticoid treatment incorporate extreme asthma, organ transplantation, cystic fibrosis, incendiary inside malady, and acceptance chemotherapy for leukemia or different malignancies.

Symptoms of Diabetes

Diabetes is an unadulterated, yet essential medicinal condition. If you have diabetes, you have to deal with your blood sugars and frequently screen them to make sure they are within their real range.

But, how can you tell that you have diabetes? Most early manifestations are from higher-than-typical levels of glucose, a sort of sugar, in your blood.

The warning symptoms can be mild to the point that you don't see them. That is particularly true, especially for type 2 diabetes. A few people don't discover they have it until the point when they get issues from long-haul harm caused by the infection.

With type 1 diabetes, the indications, for the most part, happen rapidly, in a matter of days or half a month. They're substantially more serious, as well.

Low glucose is frequent in people with type 1 and types 2 DM. Most cases are mellow and are not viewed as therapeutic crises. Impacts can extend from sentiments of unease, sweating, trembling, and expanded hunger in mellow instances to more difficult issues, for example, disarray, changes in conduct, for instance, forcefulness, seizures, obviousness, and (rarely) lasting cerebrum harm or demise in serious cases. Moderate hypoglycemia may effortlessly be mixed up for drunkenness; fast breathing and sweating, cold, fair skin are normal for hypoglycemia however not definitive. Mild to direct cases are self-treated by eating or drinking something high in sugar. Severe cases can prompt obviousness and must be treated with intravenous glucose or infusions with glucagon.

Individuals (more often than not with type 1 DM) may likewise encounter scenes of diabetic ketoacidosis, an unsettling metabolic influence portrayed by sickness, retching, and stomach torment.

They possess a scent reminiscent of CH3)2CO on the breath, deep breathing known as Kussmaul breathing, and in severe cases a diminished level of consciousness.

A rare however similarly extreme probability is a hyperosmolar hyperglycemic state, which is more common in Type 2 DM and is chiefly the consequence of parchedness.

Diabetes manifestations may happen after some time, or they may show up rapidly. The different types of diabetes may have equal or diverse cautioning signs. Some cautioning signs of diabetes are:

- Dry mouth
- Frequent urination
- Yeast infections
- Blurred vision
- Wounds that don't heal quickly
- Extreme thirst
- Hunger
- Fatigue
- Irritable behavior
- Skin that itches or is dry

CHAPTER THREE

DIABETES COMPLICATION AND PROGRESSION

Complications are problems that occur as a result of a malady. On account of diabetes, there are two sorts of complications. The first kind happens rapidly and can be managed hastily. This kind is called an intense entanglement. The other type is caused by the blood sugar being too high for a long time and is known as an unending difficulty or long haul complexity.

Overabundance blood glucose is called 'hyperglycemia.' If high, it can cause severe complications. In Type 1 diabetics, one of these complications is diabetic ketoacidosis which is a therapeutic crisis and can often be recognized by a fruity scent on the breath. Another intense difficulty, more common in Type 2 diabetics, is non-ketotic hyperosmolar extreme lethargies which are likewise exceptionally unsafe. Too low blood glucose is called hypoglycemia. It can likewise cause acute complications. Diabetics can have numerous indications, for example, sweating, trembling, outrage (or feeling uninvolved), and perhaps notwithstanding going out. People with diabetes with hypoglycemia might be confounded or even oblivious. They may seem to have drunk liquor excessively. Extreme hypoglycemia is exceptionally unsafe and can cause passing. The best treatment for hypoglycemia is maintaining a strategic distance from it. On the off chance that it happens, eating sustenance containing glucose (for instance, table sugar) more often than not enhances the condition rapidly. It is however treated by giving an infusion of a prescription called 'glucagon.'

Glucagon is a hormone created by the pancreas. It has the contrary impact of insulin. Managing glucagon will cause the blood glucose level to ascend by constraining put away glucose into the blood. Hypoglycemia is caused by an excessive amount of diabetic pharmaceutical, deficient sustenance, an excess of activity, or a mix of these.

Uncontrolled diabetes can prompt various short and long-haul wellbeing complications, including hypoglycemia, coronary illness, and vision issues.

However, the massive part of these diabetes-related conditions happen because of uncontrolled blood glucose levels, especially lifted glucose over a drawn-out timeframe. It is fundamental that diabetics are aware of the complications that can occur because of diabetes to guarantee that the main side effects of any conceivable sickness are spotted before they create.

Perpetual complications are for the most part caused by hyperglycemia (however not sufficiently high to dependably purpose serious complexities). It makes harm veins and nerves. Harm to veins can inevitably cause strokes, heart assaults, kidney disappointment, visual deficiency, moderate recuperating of skin breaks - with the included plausibility of disease - and even removals from the poor course (diminished bloodstream, for the most part to the feet and toes). Harm to nerves can make diabetics not feel torment (this, for the most part, occurs in their feet). This makes them have more wounds and not understand they have harmed themselves. Harm to nerves can likewise cause torment notwithstanding when there's no substantial damage. It's a type of apparition agony or phantom pain. The torture can be intense to the point that considerable torment prescription might be required.

Managing Diabetes complications

Given the harm caused by high blood glucose, it is vital to treat diabetes mellitus. The objective is to keep up a typical blood glucose level. The usual range for blood glucose is 80-120 mg/dL (milligrams of glucose per deciliter of blood) or 3.5-7 mmol/l (millimole per liter of blood.) These are unique methods for saying a similar thing, much like yards and meters are diverse units of separation estimation.

Diabetics (people suffering from diabetes) should check their blood sugar often. This is to ensure they don't get hypoglycemia or hyperglycemia. A glucometer is a battery fueled estimating apparatus that tests the blood sugar level. Diabetics often go along with their glucometer to monitor their sugar level or visit medical centers to check their glucose level a few times in a day. They may likewise endure severe clogging and incessant pee.

Specialists may likewise utilize a blood test called a hemoglobin A1C. This is once in a while composed Hgb-A1C or different routes; there's no standard name. This tells the specialist what the average blood glucose has been for the previous three months.

Diabetics must be checked for signs of complications because of diabetes. They should see an eye specialist consistently to be reviewed for harm to the veins in the eyes. On the off chance that this isn't found and treated early, it can cause a visual deficiency. They ought to have their pee or blood frequently checked for signs of kidney harm. They should check their feet for cuts, wounds, rankles, et cetera no less than consistently. Furthermore, they ought to have their feet frequently checked for nerves damage, circulatory issues, and diseases.

CHAPTER FOUR
UNDERSTANDING DIABETES PROGRESSION

The toll diabetes is taking over the globe is quite stunning. It is the primary source of new instances of grown-up visual impairment, final phase renal malady, and limited non-traumatic amputations.

What's more, patients with diabetes have a rate of cardiovascular morbidity and mortality four times that of non-diabetics. 65% of patients with Type 2 diabetes will kick the bucket of a cardiovascular confusion.

Fortunately, complications of diabetes can be constrained, and its movement impeded with strict control of glucose and new treatment conventions. Insulin sensitizers, insulin secretagogues, pharmaceuticals that modify the processing of sugars and further insulin details might be joined to make a synergistic impact to accomplish a glycemic target.

Nursing care should be in a state of harmony with this new assault. Medical caretakers in all settings must comprehend the importance of glycemic control and get comfortable with new treatment systems.

Our compass starts here with a discourse of Syndrome X, which many refer to as an antecedent to diabetes.

However, let's be quick to understand that the two most recurring type of diabetes is the Type 1 and 2

The contrasts between Type 1 and 2 diabetes

Diabetes is a mind-boggling jumble that influences the emission, digestion, and capacity of the hormone insulin. There are numerous types. However, Type 1 and 2 are the two most common.

In Type 1 diabetes, the insulin-creating beta cells of the pancreas are dynamically annihilated in an immune system reaction to a viral or ecological affront. In spite of the fact that the dangerous procedure might be subclinical for a considerable length of time, side effects regularly grow suddenly. Trademark signs incorporate intemperate thirst, visit pee, and expanded hunger (polydipsia, polyuria, and polyphagia), and also weight reduction.

Type 1 diabetes more often than not happens before age 40, with a pinnacle rate at age 13. However, it can create in individuals as youthful as 1 or as old as 70. An individual may have hereditary powerlessness to the affront that triggers the invulnerable framework reaction, yet there's no substantial genetic segment to the sickness itself.

Over 80% of all diabetics have Type 2 diabetes. Type 2 is a muddle up of three fundamental issues: insulin protection, beta cell destruction, and expanded glucose creation by the liver. The malady regularly starts in middle age or later, with most individuals creating it in their 60s. However, there has been an emotional increment in the number of kids who are creating Type 2 diabetes.

Patients are frequently indication free for up to six years previously analysis. At that point, noteworthy organ harm is now present – 20% will have retinopathy. Although the main reason for the metabolic imperfections included isn't known, we do realize that there is a reliable hereditary connection. For instance, Type 2 diabetes is discovered all the more much of the time in certain ethnic gatherings. Now there's additionally new proof connecting fetal and baby sustenance to the metabolic changes that prompt Type 2 diabetes.

Diabetes starts with insulin Tolerance

Insulin tolerance is a cell resistance to the action of insulin on both skeletal muscles and fat cells, which impedes the take-up of glucose. The body perceives that tissues aren't getting the glucose they need and tries to remunerate by delivering more insulin, bringing about hyperinsulinemia.

Most individuals' beta cells can't stay aware of the interest for more insulin on a long haul premise, however. So insulin emission reductions and in the first place, there'll be a transient rise in glucose after dinners – when there's an expansion in the material to be utilized – , and afterward, as the beta cells keep on failing, a condition of persevering hyperglycemia will result.

The blend of insulin Tolerance and a mellow modification in beta cell work prompts hindered glucose resilience. The American Diabetes Association characterizes IGT as a fasting serum glucose <126 mg/dL, and a serum glucose > 140 mg/dL yet < 200 mg/dL two hours after a 75 mg glucose challenge. Just a single out of four patients with disabled glucose resistance will advance to Type 2 diabetes. Therefore, clinicians used to give careful consideration to IGT other than to take note of that it was a pre-diabetic condition.

In spite of the fact that an inclination for insulin Tolerance is acquired, heftiness and an inactive way of life quicken its movement toward

IGT and Type 2 diabetes.3 One examination showed that 20% expanded the danger of insulin Tolerance Syndrome for each 5% put on in weight from age 20 to age 53.5 Now we see this hazard increment among school-age youngsters, also.

Individuals with disabled glucose resilience do, however, tend to display a bunch of irregularities that respond synergistically and have come to be alluded to as insulin Tolerance Syndrome or, essentially, Syndrome X: hyperinsulinemia, hypertension, hypertriglyceridemia, low levels of HDL cholesterol, and an adjustment in size and thickness of LDL cholesterol. Most of the inconvenience starts with a lot of insulin.

Taking excess of insulin-induced recipe is as terrible as having little of it

Insulin progresses glucose take-up, as well as attempts to take abundance glucose and transform it into fat – triglycerides, to be correct. Insulin additionally advances fat stockpiling, smothers protein breakdown, and helps protein union. The compensatory ascend in insulin caused by a Tolerance from it prompts elevated amounts of unsaturated fats in the blood that are in the long run put away in fat tissue, especially in the abdomen.

Surplus insulin likewise causes the kidneys to cling to sodium and decreases their capacity to dispose of uric corrosive, which prompts hypertension and hyperuricemia. It additionally influences vascular endothelial cells to venture up a group of plasminogen activator inhibitor-1 (PAI-1), which keeps the breakdown of clumps and prompts microthrombi and endothelial inflammation.

Hyperinsulinemia meddles with intracellular pH and calcium fixation, which increments vascular tone and upgrades vasoconstriction.7 Excess insulin additionally advances a move in LDL cholesterol from a considerable molecule to one with bringing down mass, making little, thick LDL particles. What's more, it diminishes HDL – the "good" cholesterol.

The substantial connection amongst hyperinsulinemia and coronary illness has made a few specialists propose that fasting insulin levels are a free hazard factor for the ischemic coronary disease. Amusingly, patients with what cardiologists have been calling Syndrome X – patients with angina, a positive pressure test, and angiographically regular coronary supply routes – likewise have hyperinsulinemia.

This significant effect on the cardiovascular framework has driven the American Heart Association to suggest changing the name insulin Tolerance Syndrome to cardiovascular dysmetabolic Syndrome. The indicative criteria incorporate dyslipidemia, insulin Tolerance, stoutness, and hypertension (DROP).

Syndrome X:

Syndrome X is currently considered a piece of an interminable second rate provocative process that advances endothelial brokenness. It quickens with age and heftiness, offering to ascend to atheromatous plaque arrangement, ischemic coronary illness, left ventricular hypertrophy, and, now and again, Type 2-diabetes. Sadly, there are no conspicuous signs and symptoms.

Screening fasting insulin isn't prescribed because there is no standard method to gauge it, and the mean level that constitutes insulin resistance has not been determined. There are a few markers of endothelial reactivity; however, there is no research facility that can recognize it.

Of course, the cardiovascular dysmetabolic disorder has turned into an essential territory of clinical research. Real endeavors now are being made to decide the ideal approach to distinguish the disease, and whether early mediation will change the movement to diabetes and additionally the advancement of cardiovascular complications.

Tight glycemic control is the way to avoidance

The American Diabetes Association guidelines released about a year ago suggest examination fasting plasma glucose and glycosylated hemoglobin (HbA1c) – the normal blood glucose level in the course of the most recent two months – to assess general glycemic control. They recommend continuing fasting glucose < 126 mg/dL and the HbA1c < 7.0%.10 Patients like Ms. Alvarez are encouraged to visit their doctor at regular intervals to survey HbA1c and keep estimating fasting glucose every morning when they wake up.

Recent corroboration shows a connection between postprandial hyperglycemia and a considerable lot of the real complications of diabetes, including retinopathy, nephropathy, and cardiovascular malady. This urges us to make blood glucose observing a stride further: Checking postprandial blood glucose can give a superior picture of general glycemic control than a fasting level and delineates how well a patient handles the everyday highs and lows, which don't show up in HbA1c.

Since patients are more frequently in a postprandial state instead of in a fasting state, wide vacillations in blood glucose for the day make them more hyperglycemic than not. Current reasoning proposes checking and all the more strongly managing blood glucose levels at mealtimes to accomplish better glycemic control for the day. The postprandial blood glucose target level is 160 mg/dL.

CHAPTER FIVE

REVERSING DIABETES

Endeavors to forestall or cure Type 1 diabetes are coordinated at anticipating or abating the immune system reaction that triggers it. Islet cell transfer is an energizing and promising area of research.

Stemming Type 2 diabetes and the broken metabolic disorder that produces cardiovascular ailment will request that we recognize those in danger, teach them about infection and way of life changes, and create compelling treatment gets ready for the individuals who already have the sickness. The objective is to keep the illness, or if nothing else moderate movement.

Most specialists, dietitians, and diabetes pros assert that type 2 diabetes is a constant and dynamic infection. When you get the conclusion, it's lifelong incarceration. It's an extraordinary enormous lie. Type 2 diabetes is almost invariably reversible, and this is virtually absurdly simple to demonstrate. Perceiving this fact is the crucial initial phase in switching your diabetes or pre-diabetes. It's something that most individuals already instinctually perceived to be valid.

Other pharmaceuticals, for example, metformin or the DPP4 tranquilize class is weight unbiased. While this won't exacerbate the situation, they won't improve things either. Since weight reduction is the way to switching Type 2-diabetes, Medications or let us say constant usage of drugs won't improve things. Pharmaceuticals make blood sugars (the side effect) better, yet not diabetes (the real ailment).

We've imagined that the manifestation is the disease.

The fundamental element of type 2 diabetes and pre-diabetes is that our bodies are filled with sugar. It's not simply an excess of sugar in the blood. That is just piece of the issue. There's a lot of sugar in our whole body. Envision our bodies to be a sugar bowl. A bowl of sugar. When we are youthful, our sugar bowl is unfilled. Over decades, we overeat of the wrong things – sugary oats, pastries, and white bread. The sugar bowl progressively tops off with sugar until full. Whenever you eat, sugar comes into the body, since the bowl is full, so it spills out into the blood.

The big question is: Why does this really happen? The answer to that is that the cells are already over-filled with glucose

The cell opposes the glucose since it's full. Insulin restraint is an *overflow conjecture.*

Be that as it may, metformin does not dispose of the sugar. Preferably, it takes the sugar from the blood and smashes it once more into the liver. The liver doesn't need it either, so it ships it out to the various organs – the kidneys, the nerves, the eyes, the heart. Quite a bit of this additional sugar will likewise simply get transformed into fat.

The issue, apparently, has not been solved – the sugar bowl is as yet overflowing. You've just moved sugar from the blood (where you could see it) into the body (where you couldn't see it). It's putting a band-help over a shot opening. Along these lines, the precise next time you eat, precisely the same happens. Sugar comes in, spills out into the blood, and you take the solution to pack the sugar once more into the body. This works for some time, yet in the long run, the body tops off with sugar, as well.

Presently, that same dosage of prescription can't compel any more sugar into the body.

Somehow the prescription seems to be working, however just for a period. Blood sugars go down as you drive your body to choke down significantly more sugar. In the long run, this dosage flops too. So then your specialist gives you a moment medicine, then a third one and afterward in the end insulin infusions.

How to Reverse Diabetes to live a healthy life

There are exceptionally just two approaches to dispose of the unnecessary sugar in the body.

Avoid too much sugar

Dispose of it completely

That is it. That is all we have to do. And the best part is? It's all regular and entirely free. No medications. No surgery. No cost.

Stage 1 – Don't place sugar in

The initial step is to dispense with all sugar and refined starches from your eating routine. Sugar has no wholesome esteem and can, therefore, be disposed of. Carbohydrates are mainly long chains of sugars. Profoundly refined polysaccharides, for example, flour or white rice are immediately separated by assimilation into glucose. This is quickly retained into the blood and raises glucose. For instance, eating white bread expands blood sugars rapidly. Doesn't it appear to be undeniable that we ought to maintain a strategic distance from sustenances that raise blood sugars since they will, in the long run, be assimilated into the body? The ideal methodology is to eat next to zero refined sugars. In particular, stick to consuming entire, regular, natural nourishment.

Stage 2 – Burn it off

Fasting is the least complicated and quickest strategy to constrain your body to consume sugar for vitality. Glucose in the blood is the most efficiently open wellspring of energy for the body. Fasting is merely the other side of eating – if you are not eating you are fasting. When you eat, your body stores sustenance vitality and when you fast, your body consumes nourishment vitality. On the off chance that you radically lengthen out your times of fasting, you can consume off the putaway sugar.

Since type 2 diabetes is simply unreasonable glucose in the body, consuming it off will invert the infection. While it might sound dangerous, fasting has been drilled for no less than 2000 years. It is the most seasoned dietary therapy known. Indeed a large number of individuals all through humanity's history have fasted without issues. If you are taking resourcefully prescribed pharmaceuticals, you should look for the persuasion of a doctor. Be that as it may, the main problem results in these present circumstances.

If you don't eat, will your blood sugars descend? And if you eat will you get more fit? Obviously.

We can turn around type 2 diabetes and pre-diabetes today, at present, promptly. All without cost, without drugs, without surgery, with an all normal, time-tried recuperating technique. We just need to lead our bodies down the recuperating pathway and have the grit to apply our hard-won learning. Type 2 diabetes is reversible. Thus the dawn of new hope for Diabetics.

Notwithstanding controlling blood glucose level, other medicines might be required. Diabetics frequently have vein infections, so it is critical to focus on other ailments which may influence veins. In individuals with diabetes, treating (hypertension) and elevated cholesterol is essential than expected and sadly, both of these maladies harm the veins. The treatment objectives can change for diabetics. For example, in individuals without diabetes, pulse ought to be 140/90 or less. In people with diabetes, it ought to be 130/80 or less.

CONCLUSION

Thank you once again for purchasing this book!

I hope you've been able to learn quite some things about diabetes, the types and most importantly how to reverse from this book.

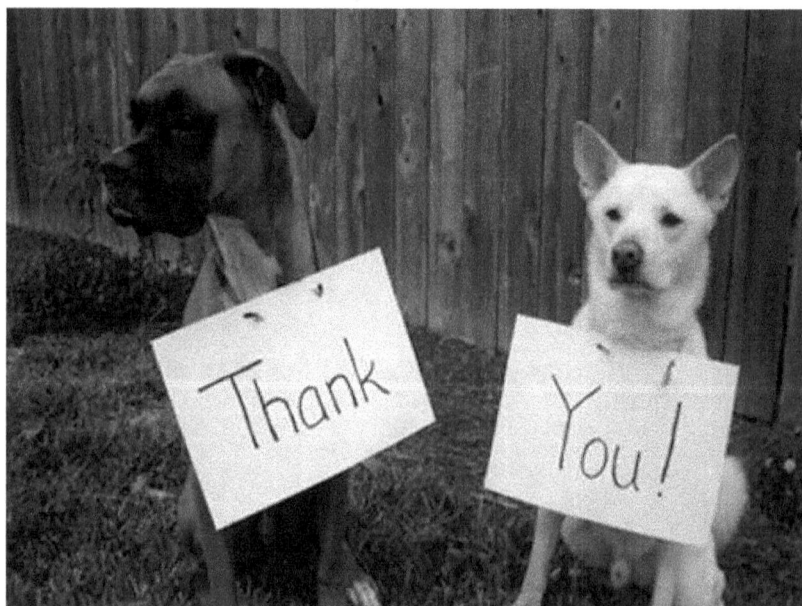

Finally, if you enjoyed this book, then I will like to ask you for a favor, would you be kind enough to leave a review for this book on Amazon? It will be greatly appreciated.

Thank You and Goodluck

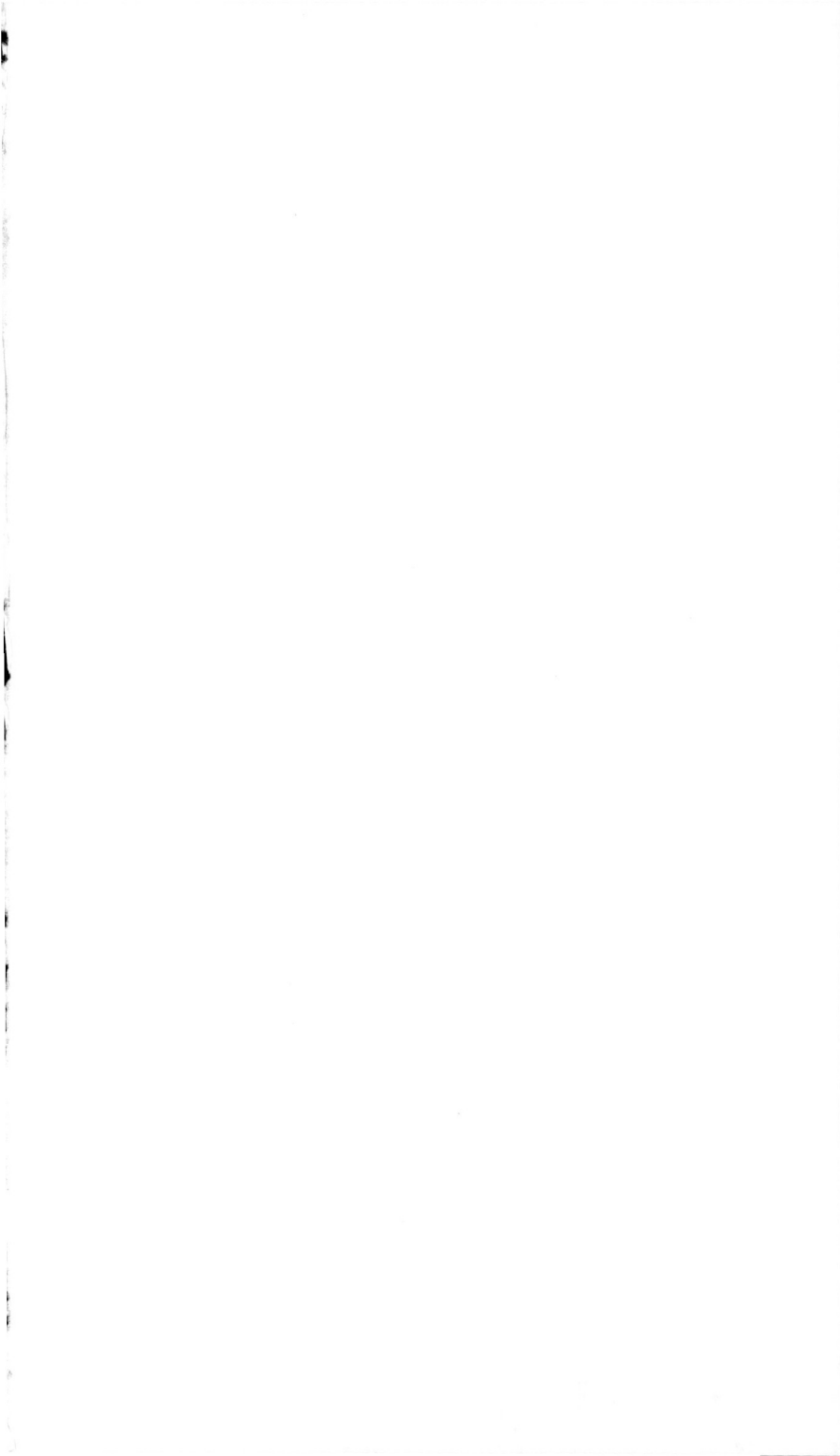